About the NCCN Guidelines for Patients®

National Comprehensive Cancer Network®

AF702065

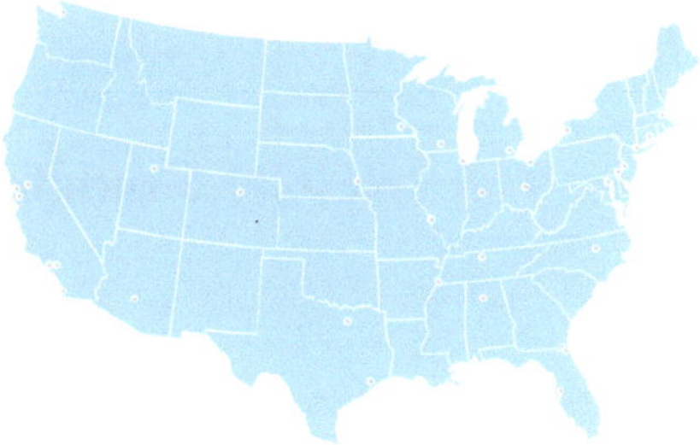

Did you know that top cancer centers across the United States work together to improve cancer care? This alliance of leading cancer centers is called the National Comprehensive Cancer Network® (NCCN®).

Cancer care is always changing. NCCN develops evidence-based cancer care recommendations used by health care providers worldwide. These frequently updated recommendations are the NCCN Clinical Practice Guidelines in Oncology (NCCN Guidelines®). The NCCN Guidelines for Patients plainly explain these expert recommendations for people with cancer and caregivers.

These NCCN Guidelines for Patients are based on the NCCN Clinical Practice Guidelines in Oncology (NCCN Guidelines®) for Anal Carcinoma, Version 4.2025 — May 30, 2025.

Learn how the NCCN Guidelines for Patients are developed
NCCN.org/patient-guidelines-process

View the NCCN Guidelines for Patients free online
NCCN.org/patientguidelines

Find an NCCN Cancer Center near you
NCCN.org/cancercenters

Connect with us

Supporters

NCCN Guidelines for Patients are supported by funding from the NCCN Foundation®

NCCN Foundation gratefully acknowledges the following corporate supporter for helping to make available these NCCN Guidelines for Patients: Taiho Oncology, Inc.

NCCN independently adapts, updates, and hosts the NCCN Guidelines for Patients. Our corporate supporters do not participate in the development of the NCCN Guidelines for Patients and are not responsible for the content and recommendations contained therein.

Fight Colorectal Cancer (Fight CRC) is a leading patient-empowerment and advocacy organization providing balanced and objective information on colon and rectal cancer research, treatment, and policy. We are relentless champions of hope, focused on funding promising, high-impact research endeavors while equipping advocates to influence legislation and policy for the collective good. Get fast answers from ChatCRC, the first and only AI chatbot for colorectal cancer by texting (318) 242-8272 or visiting chatbot.fightcrc.org. For ways to join the fight, visit FightCRC.org.

To make a gift or learn more, visit online or email

NCCNFoundation.org/Donate

PatientGuidelines@NCCN.org

Contents

NCCN Foundation seeks to support the millions of patients and their families affected by a cancer diagnosis by funding and distributing NCCN Guidelines for Patients. NCCN Foundation is also committed to advancing cancer treatment by funding the nation's promising doctors at the center of innovation in cancer research. For more details and the full library of patient and caregiver resources, visit NCCN.org/patients.

National Comprehensive Cancer Network (NCCN) and NCCN Foundation
3025 Chemical Road, Suite 100, Plymouth Meeting, PA 19462 USA

1
About anal cancer

Treatment for anal cancer should involve a team of digestive health experts with experience in chemotherapy, radiation therapy, surgery, and imaging. Everyone with anal cancer is encouraged to enroll in a clinical trial for treatment, when possible.

What is anal cancer?

The anus is the opening at the end of the large intestine through which feces (stool) leaves the body. Anal cancer starts in either the **anal canal** or the **perianal region**.

The **anal canal** is about the length of a paper clip and connects the rectum and the anal opening. Most anal cancers start here, in cells called squamous cells. Cancer that forms in squamous cells is called squamous cell carcinoma.

The **perianal region (also called the anal margin)** includes the anal opening and the skin directly surrounding it. In some cases, an anal tumor can involve both the anal canal and the perianal skin.

Anal squamous cell carcinoma is the focus of this resource. Other rare types of anal cancer not covered here include anal adenocarcinoma and anal melanoma. NCCN Guidelines for Patients are available on these topics.

The anus

Anal cancer starts in either the anal canal or the perianal region. The anal canal connects the rectum and the anal opening. The perianal region includes the anal opening and the skin directly surrounding it.

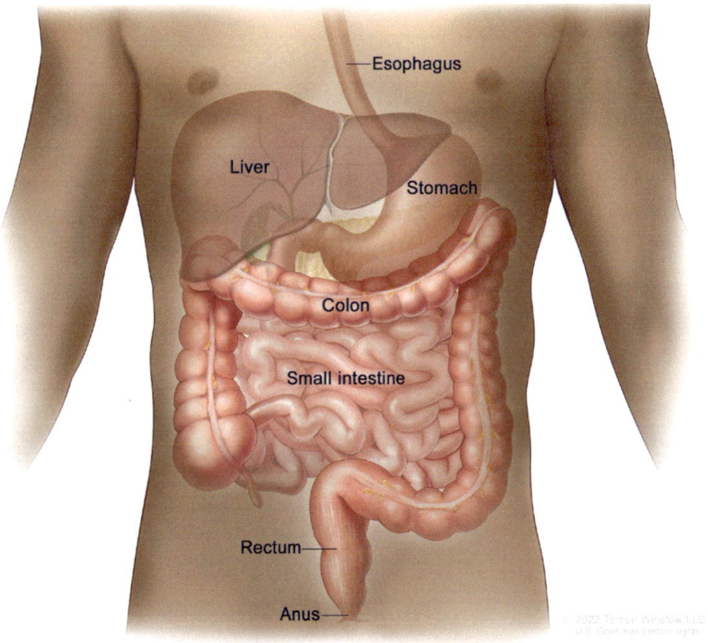

Who is at risk for anal cancer?

A risk factor is something that increases the risk of developing a disease. Some people with no known risk factors will develop anal cancer, while others with risk factors will not.

HPV infection

The risk factor most strongly linked with anal cancer is long-term infection with human papillomavirus (HPV). HPV is the most common sexually transmitted virus. It affects almost everyone who has ever been sexually active. Most people are unaware that they are (or ever were) infected.

In most people, the immune system gets rid of HPV from the body. But in some people the virus causes long-term cell changes that develop into cancer, often decades after the initial infection. Cancers caused by HPV include anal, cervical, head and neck, penile, vaginal, and vulvar cancers.

There are more than 100 types (called strains) of HPV. Infection with some strains is more likely to lead to anal cancer and related cancers. High-risk strains include HPV-16 and HPV-18. HPV infection can also cause abnormal skin growths, called warts, to form on the anus or genitals.

A vaccine that protects against 9 different strains of HPV, including the highest-risk strains, is available. Vaccination is recommended for all adolescents and young adults, and is an option for adults aged 45 or below. The vaccine is most effective in younger people because they have likely never been exposed to HPV.

Guide 1 Risk factors for anal cancer
Long-term HPV infection
HIV infection
Taking anti-rejection medicines after an organ transplant
Cervical, vulvar, or vaginal cancer or pre-cancer
Anal pre-cancer
Blood cancers, such as lymphoma, chronic lymphocytic leukemia, or multiple myeloma
Tobacco use
Anal sex
Other sexually transmitted infections
Autoimmune disorders, such as Crohn's disease

Other risk factors

Health conditions and other factors that increase the risk of anal cancer are listed in **Guide 1.** Some of these increase risk because they weaken the immune system, making it harder for the body to clear HPV infection.

How does anal cancer start?

Anal cancer starts as areas of abnormal cells, called lesions, in or near the anus. These pre-cancerous lesions are known as anal dysplasia.

Identifying and treating anal dysplasia may prevent anal cancer. Other names for anal dysplasia include:

- Low-grade squamous intraepithelial lesion (LSIL), which is mild dysplasia
- High-grade squamous intraepithelial lesion (HSIL), which is moderate or severe dysplasia
- Anal intraepithelial neoplasia (AIN)
- Stage 0 anal cancer

What can I do to get the best care?

Advocate for yourself. You have an important role to play in your care. In fact, you're more likely to get the care you want by asking questions and making shared decisions with your care team.

The NCCN Guidelines for Patients will help you understand cancer care. With better understanding, you'll be more prepared to discuss your care with your team and share your concerns. Many people feel more satisfied when they play an active role in their care.

Why you should read this book

Making decisions about cancer care can be stressful. You may need to make tough decisions under pressure about complex choices.

The NCCN Guidelines for Patients are trusted by patients and providers. They clearly explain current care recommendations made by respected experts in the field. Recommendations are based on the latest research and practices at leading cancer centers.

Cancer care is not the same for everyone. By following expert recommendations for your situation, you are more likely to improve your care and have better outcomes as a result. Use this book as your guide to find the information you need to make important decisions.

You may not know what to ask your care team. That's common. Each chapter in this book ends with an important section called *Questions to ask*. These suggested questions will help you get more information on all aspects of your care.

Take the next step and keep reading to learn what is the best care for you!

2
Testing for anal cancer

This chapter describes the testing and care needed to diagnose anal cancer and create your treatment plan.

First steps

The most common symptom of anal cancer is bleeding from the anus, also called rectal bleeding. You may notice blood in your stool, on toilet paper, or in the water of the toilet bowl. Anal itching is also common. Some people have pain in the anal area or feel like there is a lump or mass near the anus.

These symptoms shouldn't be ignored. It's common to assume they are caused by hemorrhoids. Although they may be embarrassing to talk about, it's important to be evaluated by a health care professional.

People with these symptoms often reach out to their primary care provider, gynecologist, or gastroenterologist. While this is an important first step, certain specialists are best qualified to evaluate you.

This includes colorectal surgeons and health care providers trained to conduct a test called high-resolution anoscopy (HRA). HRA typically takes place after a digital rectal exam (DRE) is performed.

Guide 2
Testing and care for anal cancer

Necessary tests	• Anoscopy • Biopsy • Digital rectal exam • Groin exam for swollen lymph nodes • To see the extent of cancer in and near the anus: Either CT or MRI • To look for cancer outside the pelvis: CT of your chest and abdomen
Other tests or care you may receive	• PET/CT or PET/MRI scan • *DPYD* testing • HIV blood test (encouraged) • Help to quit smoking • Gynecologic exam including screening for cervical cancer • Fertility preservation

Digital rectal exam

The digital rectal exam (DRE) is important for diagnosis, staging, and follow-up. In a DRE, your doctor inserts a gloved, lubricated finger into your anus and rectum. This finger exam can find abnormalities in the anal canal and nearby areas.

High-resolution anoscopy

High-resolution anoscopy (HRA) is a procedure that allows your health care provider to view and examine the anal canal with magnification.

After applying a numbing gel to the anal area, your provider will insert a short, hollow tool (an anoscope) a few inches into the anus. Next, they will apply a liquid called acetic acid to the anal canal tissue. Using a special magnifying glass called a colposcope, they will closely examine the tissues of the anal canal. The acetic acid makes abnormal cells stand out when viewed with the colposcope.

If your provider sees any abnormal or suspicious areas, they will remove a sample of tissue for testing. This is called a biopsy. This biopsy sample may provide the diagnosis of anal cancer. If a colposcope *isn't* used for the procedure, it's called standard anoscopy. HRA may be more effective than standard anoscopy at identifying anal cancer and pre-cancer.

No special preparations need to be taken ahead of HRA. The procedure is brief (about 20 to 30 minutes), generally painless, and you can go home afterward. Some people have minor bleeding and discomfort for a few days following the procedure. While not common, some people may need to have HRA in the operating room under general anesthesia.

SISCCA

Superficially invasive squamous cell carcinoma (SISCCA) is the earliest form of anal cancer. These lesions are smaller than a pea and not deep at all. They are often found by chance during a biopsy, or during removal of growths thought to be non-cancerous.

If the lesion is completely removed during surgery, you may be done with treatment. However, close follow-up that includes HRA is needed to check for cancer in and near the anus, including the closest lymph nodes.

This resource applies to treatment of invasive anal cancer diagnosed by biopsy and found to be more advanced than SISCCA.

Testing after diagnosis

After a biopsy confirms anal squamous cell carcinoma, more testing is needed to plan your treatment. Digital rectal exams are repeated, along with the tests described next.

Lymph node exam

There are hundreds of small bean-shaped filters in the body, called lymph nodes. These immune system helpers catch and remove things that don't belong, including cancer cells.

Certain areas of the body, like the groin, contain more lymph nodes than others. Lymph nodes in the groin are called the **inguinal** lymph nodes. If left untreated, the cancer cells can travel through blood or lymph to the inguinal or other nodes in the pelvis, and then to other areas of the body.

Lymph nodes can't usually be seen or felt in the early stages of cancer, but may become enlarged in later stages. Your provider will examine lymph nodes in your groin by pressing on the surface of the skin. This is called palpation.

If any lymph nodes feel enlarged or look suspicious on imaging tests, you may have fine-needle aspiration (FNA). For FNA, a health care provider uses a thin needle to remove a sample of tissue from the node(s) for testing.

In some cases, all or part of a lymph node may need to be removed by cutting into the skin. This is called an excisional biopsy.

Imaging

Imaging tests provide information on how much cancer is in the body and where it's located. To see the extent of cancer in the anus and nearby areas (including lymph nodes), either computed tomography (CT)

Imaging

To see the extent of cancer in the anus and nearby, either a CT or MRI scan is recommended. CT uses a small amount of radiation to create images; MRI uses magnetic fields.

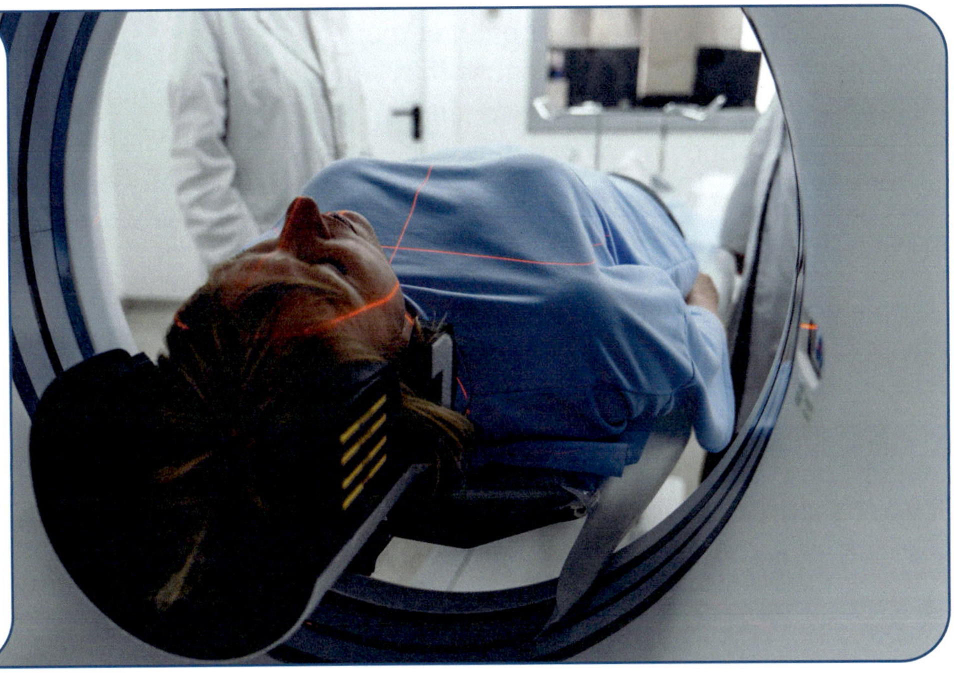

or magnetic resonance imaging (MRI) is recommended.

Both types of scanners are large machines with tunnel-like openings in the middle. While the process is similar, MRI takes longer and the scanner is more enclosed.

MRI doesn't use radiation and is safe for most people. Those with certain heart monitors, pacemakers, or some types of surgical clips generally can't have MRI scanning.

For either type of scan, you are likely to receive a contrast agent to make the pictures clearer. It may be given as a drink, injected into your vein, or both. In some people, contrast causes an allergic reaction. Tell your provider if you've had an issue with contrast in the past.

To look for areas of cancer beyond the pelvis, a CT scan of your chest and abdomen (with contrast) is recommended.

In some cases, positron emission tomography (PET) may be combined with CT or MRI. In a PET scan, cancer cells appear brighter than normal cells. This happens because they react differently to a radioactive glucose (sugar) that is put into your body beforehand.

HIV testing

People with HIV are at increased risk of developing anal cancer. It's good to know your HIV status. If you haven't been tested, your provider may recommend an HIV blood test.

If you have HIV, getting the care you need may also improve your cancer treatment outcomes.

Gynecologic exam

Like anal cancer, HPV is the cause of almost all cervical cancers. A gynecologic exam, including screening for cervical cancer, is recommended.

Cervical cancer screening involves scraping cells from the cervix and testing them for HPV, cancer, and cell changes that may lead to cancer. If testing for HPV isn't performed, it's simply called a Pap test. If the cells are tested for both HPV and cancer, it's called an HPV/ Pap co-test.

DPYD testing

Capecitabine and fluorouracil (5-FU) are chemotherapy medicines called fluoropyrimidines. They are commonly used to treat anal cancer. Your body uses a special enzyme (protein) called DPD to break down these medicines so they can work properly and safely.

Around 1 in 15 people inherit a difference in the gene involved in making DPD, the *DPYD* gene. This is called DPD deficiency. In these people, fluoropyrimidines can build up and cause severe and sometimes life-threating side effects, referred to as fluoropyrimidine toxicity.

Signs and symptoms include mouth sores, abdominal pain, blood in the stool, nausea, vomiting, and diarrhea. The skin on the palms of your hands and soles of your feet may start peeling and become red, swollen, or numb. Other possible side effects include shortness of breath and hair loss.

Genetic testing can be performed to learn if you have the gene variant (difference) that causes DPD deficiency. If treatment with a fluoropyrimidine is planned, talk to your provider about the risk for fluoropyrimidine toxicity. After understanding your risk, you may choose to have genetic testing for *DPYD* variants.

If you develop any of the symptoms mentioned above in the days after receiving capecitabine or 5-FU, contact your care team right away. There is an FDA-approved treatment for this uncommon side effect of fluoropyrimidines.

Staging

The results of testing are used to determine the cancer stage. The stage describes the extent of cancer in the body. The tumor, node, metastasis (TNM) system is used to stage anal squamous cell carcinomas.

Three key pieces of information are used to determine the stage:

T: The size and extent of invasion of the anal tumor. Tumors are measured in centimeters (cm). Approximately 2 and a half cm make up one inch.

N: Whether any lymph nodes near the anus have cancer

M: Whether the cancer has metastasized (spread) to areas far from the anus, such as the liver or lungs

It's important for the cancer to be staged accurately. This helps determine the best treatment plan for you. It also suggests how likely the cancer is to be cured using current treatments.

Precancer

There are abnormal cells on the surface of the anal canal or perianal region. These lesions may develop into cancer. Treatment may involve close monitoring, electrocautery by an HRA provider, or surgical removal. Names for anal precancer include:

- stage 0 anal cancer
- anal dysplasia
- carcinoma in situ
- high-grade anal intraepithelial neoplasia (AIN)
- high-grade squamous intraepithelial lesions (HSIL)

Stage 1

In stage 1 anal cancer, the tumor is 2 cm or smaller. Cancer hasn't spread to nearby lymph nodes or to areas far from the anus. Stage 1 anal cancer is described as T1, N0, M0.

Stage 2

Stage 2 anal cancer is divided into 2 substages, depending on the size of the tumor.

Anal tumors larger than 2 cm but not larger than 5 cm are stage 2A. This stage is described as T2, N0, M0.

Anal tumors larger than 5 cm are stage 2B. This stage is described as T3, N0, M0.

Stage 2 anal cancers haven't spread to nearby lymph nodes or to areas far from the anus.

Stage 3

In stage 3, there may be cancer in nearby lymph nodes. This stage has 3 sub-stages.

In stage 3A, the anal tumor is 5 cm or smaller and there is cancer in nearby lymph nodes. This stage is described as either T1, N1, M0 or T2, N1, M0.

In stage 3B, the tumor has invaded nearby organs (such as the vagina, urethra, or bladder), but there is no cancer in nearby lymph nodes. This stage is described as T4, N0, M0.

In stage 3C, the tumor is larger than 5 cm or has invaded nearby organs. Cancer has spread to nearby lymph nodes. This stage is described as either T3, N1, M0 or T4, N1, M0.

Stage 4

The cancer is metastatic. This means it has spread to areas beyond the pelvis, such as the liver or lungs. Stage 4 anal cancer is described as T (may be 1, 2, 3, or 4), N (0 or 1), M1.

Staging and treatment

Stages 1, 2, and 3 anal cancer are non-metastatic. This means they haven't spread to distant areas of the body. Because these stages are potentially curable, the goal of treatment is to cure the cancer.

Aside from some early-stage perianal cancers, treatment with chemoradiation is recommended for most non-metastatic anal cancers, regardless of the stage.

The main treatment for metastatic anal cancer, in contrast, is chemotherapy or immunotherapy. The goal of treatment for metastatic anal cancer is usually to help you live longer and to help with symptoms.

Detailed treatment information is provided in the next chapter.

Fertility and family planning

Treatment for anal cancer, especially radiation therapy, can impair your ability to have children.

Radiation damages the ovaries and testicles, causing them to stop making hormones needed for natural pregnancy. In some cases, treatment with chemotherapy can also impair fertility by damaging sperm or eggs.

If you want the option of having children after treatment or are unsure, tell your care team. They can explain any fertility-related risks of your treatment plan.

You can also ask for a referral to an expert to learn about options for preserving your fertility, including those described next.

Sperm banking

Sperm banking stores semen for later use by freezing it in liquid nitrogen.

Egg freezing

Like sperm banking, unfertilized eggs can be removed, frozen, and stored for later use.

Ovarian tissue banking

This method involves removing part or all of an ovary and freezing the part that contains the eggs. The frozen tissue that contains the eggs can later be unfrozen and put back in the body.

Ovarian transposition

This procedure moves one or both ovaries and fallopian tubes out of the range of the radiation beam. Another name for this procedure is oophoropexy.

For more information on this topic, see the *NCCN Guidelines for Patients: Adolescent and Young Adult Cancer* at NCCN.org/patientguidelines and on the NCCN Patient Guides for Cancer app.

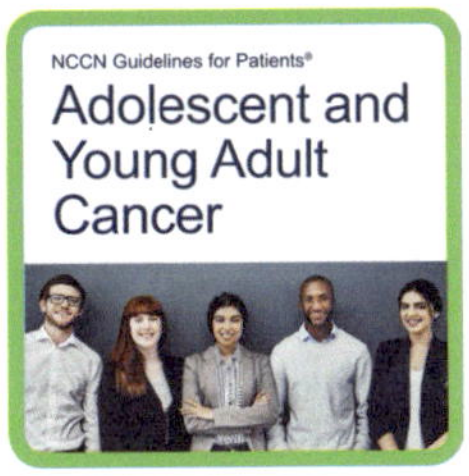

Key points

- After a biopsy confirms anal squamous cell carcinoma, more testing is needed to plan your treatment.
- Other recommended care includes a digital rectal exam (DRE), lymph node exam, imaging, HIV blood test, and screening for cervical cancer.
- After understanding your risk for fluoropyrimidine toxicity, you may choose to have testing for gene variants that cause DPD deficiency.
- The results of testing are used to determine the cancer stage. Stages 1, 2, and 3 are non-metastatic. Stage 4 is metastatic.
- Treatment for anal cancer can impair your fertility. If you want the option of having children or are unsure, talk to your care team about ways to preserve your fertility.

Questions to ask

- Did I have high-resolution anoscopy? If I didn't, will I?
- What type of anal cancer do I have? How do you know?
- What is the cancer stage?
- What is the cancer grade? What does this mean?
- Will I have any genetic tests?

3 Treatment for anal cancer

Treatment with chemoradiation is recommended for most non-metastatic anal cancers. Metastatic anal cancer is treated with a combination of chemotherapy and immunotherapy.

Anal canal cancer (stages 1 to 3)

This section provides treatment recommendations for stage 1, 2, and 3 anal canal cancers. These stages are non-metastatic, meaning the cancer hasn't spread beyond the pelvis.

Treatment with chemoradiation, described next, is recommended for all stage 1 to 3 squamous cell carcinomas in the anal canal. This combined treatment approach involves both chemotherapy and radiation therapy given during the same time period.

Chemoradiation

Radiation therapy

In external radiation therapy, radiation is delivered using a large machine outside the body. The radiation passes through skin and other tissue to reach the tumor. The radiation beams are shaped to the cancer site. This helps minimize damage to healthy tissue.

An advanced radiation technique called intensity-modulated radiation therapy (IMRT) is preferred for treating anal cancer. IMRT is unique because it allows a high dose of radiation to target the tumor while limiting the amount that reaches nearby areas, like your hip joints and external genitalia. This can help reduce treatment-related side effects.

As part of chemoradiation, radiation is typically given Monday through Friday for 5 to 6 weeks (25 to 30 treatment sessions). Your radiation oncologist will create a treatment plan to aim radiation beams at the anal tumor and lymph nodes in the pelvis and groin.

See page 19 for important information on the side effects of radiation therapy.

Chemotherapy

Chemotherapy is the use of anti-cancer medicines. Some chemotherapies can be taken by mouth, but most are given intravenously. This means the medicine is slowly infused into your body through a vein. It travels in the bloodstream to reach cells throughout the body.

Chemotherapy regimens currently recommended for use with radiation therapy to treat stage 1, 2, and 3 anal cancer are described in **Guide 3 on the next page.**

While you receive chemotherapy with one of these regimens, you will also have radiation therapy 5 days per week.

See page 19 for important information on the side effects of chemotherapy.

All treatments listed in this guide are recommended and appropriate. When helpful, NCCN experts also assign a level of preference to their recommendations for systemic therapies:

- **Preferred therapies** have the most evidence they may work better and may be safer than other therapies.
- **Other recommended therapies** can provide effective results but may have less evidence, more side effects, or may not work quite as well as preferred therapies.

Guide 3
Chemotherapy regimens for chemoradiation

Capecitabine and mitomycin **(a preferred regimen)**	**Capecitabine** is taken by mouth twice daily on radiation days (Monday through Friday) for 5 and a half to 6 weeks. On the day you begin taking capecitabine, you will also receive a single intravenous dose of **mitomycin**. A second dose may be needed when week 5 starts. Ask your provider how you can safely avoid the second dose.
5-FU and mitomycin **(a preferred regimen)**	**5-FU** is given by continuous infusion over several days. Before chemotherapy begins, you will have a device inserted into your upper chest, or a special IV inserted into your arm (a PICC line), that allows you to receive treatment from anywhere. The 5-FU is stored in a small, wearable pump that slowly infuses the medicine into the body. The first infusion starts when radiation therapy begins and lasts for 4 to 5 days. You will have another 4- to 5-day infusion at the start of week 5 of radiation therapy. The pump will be disconnected and removed between infusions. A single dose of **mitomycin** is given on the first day of the first 5-FU infusion. A second dose may be needed. Ask your provider how you can safely avoid the second dose.
5-FU and cisplatin **(recommended regimen)**	**5-FU** is given as described directly above. **Cisplatin** is given intravenously on the first day of 5-FU infusions.

Short-term side effects of radiation therapy

Common side effects at the treatment site during the 5 to 6 weeks of treatment include skin irritation, tenderness, redness, and sores or skin breakdown.

Talk to your radiation oncologist about over-the-counter ointments like Aquaphor or Silvadene. They can soothe the skin and help with healing.

Other short-term side effects of radiation therapy include diarrhea, fatigue, frequent urination or pain while urinating, and nausea. Most of these decrease over time when treatment is over.

Radiation therapy side effects may not be felt immediately. They can appear and worsen later in the cycle or even after it is complete.

Long-term side effects of radiation therapy

Radiation therapy for anal cancer can have long-term and potentially serious effects on fertility, sexual health, and bowel and bladder function.

Radiation damages the hormone-making function of the ovaries and testicles. This can cause the inability to conceive a child. Damage to the ovaries is known as premature ovarian insufficiency (POI) or radiation-induced premature menopause. You may need to see your gynecologist or primary care physician to discuss how to manage the symptoms of early menopause.

Radiation to the pelvic area can also cause the vagina to become shorter and narrower. This can make it uncomfortable or even painful to have sex, or to have vaginal exams by a doctor. Using a device called a vaginal dilator during and after radiation therapy can help gradually stretch and widen the vagina.

In those assigned male at birth, long-term risks to sexual function include erectile dysfunction and decreased testosterone function.

See *Chapter 4: Survivorship* for information on how to prevent or manage these effects.

Side effects of chemotherapy

The most common side effects of the recommended chemotherapy regimens are nausea, vomiting, diarrhea, sores in the mouth and lining of the anus, and low blood cell counts.

Low white blood cell counts can make you prone to infections. Your care team can help prevent or lessen the side effects of chemotherapy.

Capecitabine can cause a side effect known as hand-foot syndrome. Symptoms include redness, swelling, and pain on the palms of the hands, bottoms of the feet, or both. Sometimes blisters appear. Your dose of capecitabine may be changed at the earliest signs of hand-foot syndrome.

Perianal cancer (stages 1 to 3)

This section provides treatment recommendations for stage 1, 2, and 3 perianal (also called anal margin) cancers. These stages are non-metastatic, meaning the cancer hasn't spread beyond the pelvis.

Like cancers in the anal canal, most perianal cancers are treated with chemoradiation. However, local excision (surgery) may be an option for some early-stage, low-risk perianal cancers. Local excision involves removing only the tumor and a small area of surrounding tissue. Lymph nodes in the pelvis aren't removed.

Local excision

Local excision is a recommended treatment option for some stage 1 and stage 2A perianal cancers. Stage 1 and 2 anal cancers have not invaded nearby lymph nodes. For local excision to be an option, the cancer must not have invaded the sphincter muscle.

The cancer grade is also important when determining if local excision is an option. The cancer grade is a rating of how fast the cancer is expected to grow and spread. It's based on how abnormal the cancer cells look when viewed under a microscope. Higher scores mean that the cancer is likely to grow and spread quickly. There are 5 possible grades:

- **GX:** Grade cannot be assessed (undetermined grade)
- **G1:** Well differentiated (low grade)
- **G2:** Moderately differentiated (intermediate grade)
- **G3:** Poorly differentiated (high grade)
- **G4:** Undifferentiated (high grade)

Local excision should only be considered for low-grade (G1) and intermediate-grade (G2) perianal cancers.

The normal tissue surrounding the lesion removed during surgery is called the surgical margin. If a margin of at least 1 centimeter (cm) is removed and it doesn't contain cancer cells, you are done with treatment.

If a margin of less than 1 cm is removed or if the tissue contains cancer cells, the preferred next step is another surgery (re-excision). But, this may not be the best option if there is a risk of losing normal bowel function.

The pathology report may also note features that suggest the cancer will return after treatment, such as tumor cells in the blood vessels or lymph vessels outside of the main tumor. This is known as lymphovascular space invasion (LVSI).

Your team will review your pathology report and discuss your options and preferences for lowering the risk of recurrence and maintaining your bowel function.

Another option is radiation therapy with or without chemotherapy. If this option is planned, chemotherapy regimens used with radiation are listed in **Guide 3**.

Chemoradiation

Chemoradiation is recommended for all non-metastatic perianal cancers that don't meet the criteria for local excision. This includes:

- Fast-growing (high-grade) stage 1 and 2 cancers
- Stage 2 cancers that have invaded the sphincter
- Stage 3 cancers

Chemoradiation for perianal cancer is the same as for anal canal cancer. See page 17 for details on chemoradiation.

Follow-up and surveillance

After finishing treatment for anal cancer, you will have testing to find early signs that cancer may have returned. This is called surveillance. The following recommendations apply to cancers in the anal canal and the perianal region.

A physical exam with digital rectal examination (DRE) and anoscopy is recommended 8 to 12 weeks after completing chemoradiation to check the results of treatment. Your provider may also order imaging tests.

Depending on the results, the cancer will be assigned to one of the following categories:

- Complete remission – there are no signs of cancer in the body
- Persistent disease – cancer remains in the body but has not grown or spread
- Progressive disease – the cancer has grown or spread

Complete remission

If initial follow-up testing finds no signs of cancer, recommended surveillance going forward is shown in **Guide 4**.

In addition to surveillance testing, a range of other care is important for anal cancer survivors. See *Chapter 4: Survivorship* for more information.

Persistent disease

If cancer is found at the first follow-up exam, it doesn't mean that treatment didn't work. Some anal cancers take longer to respond to treatment than others. It may be safe to monitor the cancer for as long as 6 months after treatment to see if there is improvement. This may avoid the need for surgery to remove the anus.

If the cancer doesn't go into complete remission or gets worse, see "Progressive disease" below. If the cancer goes into remission, surveillance as described above under *Complete remission* is started.

Progressive disease

If the follow-up exam 8 to 12 weeks after treatment finds that the cancer has progressed, a biopsy will be performed to be certain.

If biopsy results confirm progression, the next step is imaging. Imaging can show if the cancer is limited to the anal area (locally progressive) or whether it has spread to areas far from the pelvis (metastatic). Surgery to remove the anus is recommended for locally progressive anal cancer. This surgery is discussed in more detail next.

Before proceeding with surgery, your provider may recommend trying immunotherapy with an immune checkpoint inhibitor. In some patients with anal cancer, immunotherapy has worked well enough that surgery hasn't been needed. However, there isn't much research available on this treatment approach. Talk to your provider about the benefits and risks of delaying surgery to try immunotherapy.

Guide 4
Surveillance for those in complete remission

• **Digital rectal exams** • **Inguinal (groin) lymph node exams**	Every 3 to 6 months for 5 years after treatment
Anoscopy	Where possible, anoscopy is recommended every 6 to 12 months for 3 years after treatment. In some people, after treatment with radiation therapy, anoscopy may not be possible due to discomfort or pain. In this case, your doctor may recommend having an exam under anesthesia. Or, you and your doctor may decide together to omit anoscopy or perform it less often than every 6 to 12 months.
Imaging	**Stage 2 and 3 cancers:** Imaging is recommended every year for 3 years. Either of the following is appropriate: • CT of your chest, abdomen, and pelvis with contrast • CT of your chest without contrast and MRI of your abdomen and pelvis with contrast

Recurrence

Recurrence is the return of cancer after a cancer-free period. Treatment depends on whether the cancer returns to the anus, to lymph nodes near the anus, or to distant areas such as the liver or lungs.

If cancer returns to the anus

If cancer returns to the anal area, surgery to remove the anus is recommended. This is called abdominoperineal resection (APR). APR is a fairly radical surgery that requires cutting into the abdomen and the perineum (the area between the anus and genitals) to remove the cancer.

In addition to the anus, APR typically involves removing the rectum, the area where the rectum and colon meet, and the fatty tissue surrounding the rectum. Lymph nodes in the groin will also be removed during surgery if any are known to have cancer.

Radiation treatment for anal cancer weakens and damages the perineum, which can interfere with healing after APR. In some cases, closing the wound requires taking tissue from another area of the body. This is known as muscle flap reconstruction. It can improve healing of the perineum and reduce complications after surgery. A muscle in the lower abdomen called the rectus abdominis, along with skin, fat, and blood vessels, is often used for reconstruction. If APR is planned, ask your provider about muscle flap reconstruction.

Removing the anus means there is no natural way for stool to exit the body. A permanent colostomy is needed. A colostomy connects the end of the colon to the outside of the abdomen. This creates an opening, called a stoma, on the surface of the abdomen. Stool exits the body through the stoma and goes into a bag attached to the skin.

Before proceeding with this radical surgery, your provider may recommend trying immunotherapy with a checkpoint inhibitor first. Sometimes immunotherapy works well enough for you to avoid surgery. But, there isn't much research available on this approach. Talk to your provider about the benefits and risks of delaying surgery to try immunotherapy.

If cancer returns to lymph nodes

Because most people have already received treatment with radiation therapy, it's generally not used again to treat the same area. In this case, a **lymph node dissection** may be needed. The lymph nodes can be dissected (removed) during APR surgery (if planned), or as a standalone procedure.

Chemotherapy is also an option for treating cancer that returns to lymph nodes in the groin. One of the following regimens is recommended:

- Carboplatin and paclitaxel
- 5-FU and cisplatin

If you didn't receive radiation therapy as part of initial treatment, it may be used to treat recurrence in groin lymph nodes. You may have chemotherapy with one of the below regimens during the same time period, as part of **chemoradiation**:

- Mitomycin and capecitabine
- 5-FU and mitomycin

Surveillance after recurrence treatment

Imaging

Imaging is recommended every year for 3 years after any type of treatment for recurrence. You may have CT of the chest, abdomen, and pelvis with contrast, or CT of the chest without contrast and an MRI of the abdomen and pelvis with contrast.

Lymph node exams

Inguinal lymph node exams are recommended every 3 to 6 months for 5 years after any type of treatment for recurrence.

Digital rectal exams

If you had treatment for cancer in lymph nodes only (you did not have APR), digital rectal exams (DREs) are recommended every 3 to 6 months for 5 years.

Anoscopy

If you had treatment for cancer in lymph nodes only (you didn't need APR), anoscopy is recommended every 6 to 12 months for 3 years.

In some people, after treatment with radiation therapy, anoscopy may not be possible due to discomfort or pain. In this case, your doctor may recommend having an exam under anesthesia. Or, you and your doctor may decide together to omit anoscopy or perform it less often than every 6 to 12 months.

Supportive care

Supportive care helps improve your quality of life during and after cancer treatment. The goal is to prevent or manage side effects and symptoms, like pain and cancer-related fatigue. It also addresses the mental, social, and spiritual concerns faced by those with cancer.

Supportive care is available to everyone with cancer and their families, not just those at the end of life. Palliative care is another name for supportive care.

Supportive care can also help with:

- ✓ Making treatment decisions
- ✓ Coordinating your care
- ✓ Paying for care
- ✓ Planning for advanced care and end of life

Metastatic anal cancer

This section provides treatment recommendations for anal cancer that has spread beyond the pelvis. If anal cancer metastasizes, it spreads most often to the liver or lungs. When possible, enrolling in a clinical trial for treatment is encouraged.

At this time, the **preferred** first-line treatment for metastatic anal cancer is a combination of platinum-based chemotherapy and immunotherapy:

- Carboplatin + paclitaxel + retifanlimab-dlwr (Zynyz)

Preferred therapies have the most evidence they may work better and may be safer than other therapies.

Other recommended options for first-line therapy are listed below. These can provide effective results but may have less evidence, more side effects, or may not work quite as well as preferred therapies:

- Carboplatin and paclitaxel
- 5-FU, leucovorin, and cisplatin (FOLFCIS)
- 5-FU, leucovorin, and oxaliplatin (mFOLFOX6)
- 5-FU and cisplatin
- Modified docetaxel, cisplatin, and fluorouracil (DCF)

After chemotherapy with certain regimens, treatment with chemoradiation may follow. Checking the extent of the cancer after chemotherapy helps guide decisions about chemoradiation.

Immunotherapy side effects

Checkpoint inhibitors have unique side effects. Unlike other cancer treatments, the side effects of immunotherapy occur because the immune system is attacking healthy cells in the body. Learning to recognize possible reactions can help you report them sooner to your care team.

More information is available at NCCN.org/patientguidelines and on the NCCN Patient Guides for Cancer app.

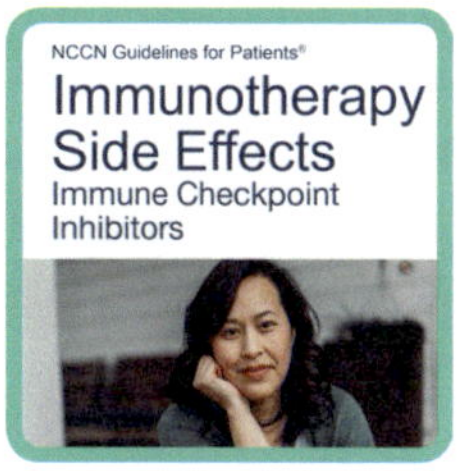

Radiation therapy

Treatment with radiation therapy (in addition to chemotherapy) is an option for newly diagnosed stage 4 anal cancers, if radiation wasn't already used. If there aren't many metastatic tumors and they are small, stereotactic body radiation therapy (SBRT) may be used.

If radiation isn't an option because the area was already treated, palliative radiation therapy can often be used to limit tumor growth and help with symptoms. If this is planned, care will be taken to ensure that areas initially treated with radiation aren't treated a second time.

Side effects of chemotherapy

The most common side effects of the chemotherapy regimens discussed above are nausea, vomiting, diarrhea, hair loss, and sores in the mouth and lining of the anus.

Platinum-based chemotherapy medicines, including carboplatin, cisplatin, and oxaliplatin, can damage the kidneys. Many people can't receive cisplatin because their kidneys don't work well or because of other health issues. To reduce the effect on the kidneys, it's common to also receive intravenous fluids.

Extended treatment with cisplatin may also cause hearing problems or hearing loss. Extended treatment with oxaliplatin can cause nerve damage to your fingers and toes. Symptoms include numbness, cramping, tingling, or pain in these areas.

Ask your care team to explain:

- How often you need to receive chemotherapy
- How long you need to receive chemotherapy
- If you will also receive immunotherapy, and for how long
- How chemotherapy or immunotherapy will be given (eg, intravenously, orally, infusion pump)

Progression

If the cancer progresses during or after treatment with chemotherapy, immunotherapy is recommended if you are eligible. Immunotherapy increases the activity of your immune system, improving your body's ability to find and destroy cancer cells. It is a type of systemic therapy.

Checkpoint inhibitors currently recommended for treating metastatic anal cancer are listed in **Guide 5**.

Guide 5
Options for immunotherapy

Generic name	Brand name
Cemiplimab-rwlc	Libtayo
Dostarlimab-gxly	Jemperli
Nivolumab	Opdivo
Pembrolizumab	Keytruda
Retifanlimab-dlwr	Zynyz
Toripalimab-pzi	Loqtorzi
Tislelizumab-jsgr	Tevimbra

Clinical trials

A clinical trial is a type of medical research study. After being developed and tested in a lab, potential new ways of fighting cancer need to be studied in people.

If found to be safe and effective in a clinical trial, a drug, device, or treatment approach may be approved by the U.S. Food and Drug Administration (FDA).

Everyone with cancer should carefully consider all of the treatment options available for their cancer type, including standard treatments and clinical trials. Talk to your doctor about whether a clinical trial may make sense for you.

Phases

Most cancer clinical trials focus on treatment and are done in phases.

- **Phase 1** trials study the safety and side effects of an investigational drug or treatment approach.
- **Phase 2** trials study how well the drug or approach works against a specific type of cancer.
- **Phase 3** trials test the drug or approach against a standard treatment. If the results are good, it may be approved by the FDA.
- **Phase 4** trials study the safety and benefit of an FDA-approved treatment.

Finding a clinical trial

In the United States

NCCN Cancer Centers
NCCN.org/cancercenters

The National Cancer Institute (NCI)
cancer.gov/about-cancer/treatment/clinical-trials/search

Worldwide

The U.S. National Library of Medicine (NLM)
clinicaltrials.gov

Need help finding a clinical trial?

NCI's Cancer Information Service (CIS)
1.800.4.CANCER (1.800.422.6237)
cancer.gov/contact

Who can enroll?

It depends on the clinical trial's rules, called eligibility criteria. The rules may be about age, cancer type and stage, treatment history, or general health. They ensure that participants are alike in specific ways and that the trial is as safe as possible for the participants.

Informed consent

Clinical trials are managed by a research team. This group of experts will review the study with you in detail, including its purpose and the risks and benefits of joining. All of this information is also provided in an informed consent form. Read the form carefully and ask questions before signing it. Take time to discuss it with people you trust. Keep in mind that you can leave and seek treatment outside of the clinical trial at any time.

Will I get a placebo?

Placebos (inactive versions of real medicines) are almost never used alone in cancer clinical trials. It's common to receive either a placebo with a standard treatment, or a new drug with a standard treatment. You will be informed, verbally and in writing, if a placebo is part of a clinical trial before you enroll.

Are clinical trials free?

There is no fee to enroll in a clinical trial. The study sponsor pays for research-related costs, including the study drug. But you may need to pay for other services, like transportation or childcare, due to extra appointments. During the trial, you will continue to receive standard cancer care. This care is often covered by insurance.

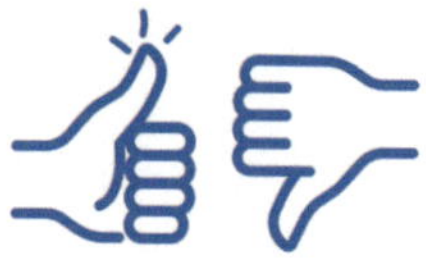

Let us know what you think!

Please take a moment to complete an online survey about the NCCN Guidelines for Patients.
NCCN.org/patients/response

Key points

- Chemoradiation is recommended for most non-metastatic cancers. The chemotherapy portion typically includes either mitomycin or 5-fluorouracil (5-FU) along with another medicine. Intensity-modulated radiation therapy (IMRT) is the preferred method.
- For some slow-growing stage 1 or 2 perianal cancers, treatment with local excision may be an option instead of chemoradiation.
- A follow-up exam with digital rectal exam (DRE) is recommended 8 to 12 weeks after completing chemoradiation to check the results of treatment.
- Surveillance during remission includes DRE, lymph node exams, and anoscopy. Yearly imaging for 3 years is also recommended for stage 2 and 3 anal cancers.
- Surgery to remove the anus may be needed for anal cancers that don't improve with initial treatment or that return afterward. It involves creating a permanent colostomy for stool to leave the body.
- If cancer returns to lymph nodes in the groin (but not to the anal area) and you had radiation as part of initial treatment, a groin dissection and/or chemotherapy is recommended.
- At this time, the preferred first-line regimen for metastatic anal cancer is a combination of platinum-based chemotherapy and immunotherapy.

Questions to ask

- Am I a candidate for surgery instead of chemoradiation?
- What are the short- and long-term side effects of chemoradiation? How can I prevent or minimize them?
- Will I have intensity-modulated radiation therapy (IMRT)?
- What happens during the simulation session?
- Will I need to take steps to ensure the safety of others in my household after radiation therapy?

4
Survivorship

Survivorship begins on the day you learn you have anal cancer. It focuses on the physical, emotional, and financial issues unique to cancer survivors.

Anal cancer survivors may experience both short- and long-term health effects of cancer and its treatment. These effects are different for everyone and depend on the treatments received.

Your primary care provider

After finishing cancer treatment, your oncologist and primary care provider should work together to provide recommended follow-up care. Ask your oncologist for a survivorship care plan that includes:

- A summary of your cancer treatment history
- A description of possible short- and long-term side effects
- Recommendations for monitoring for recurrence
- Clear roles and responsibilities for your providers
- Recommendations on your overall health and well-being

Late and long-term side effects

Some side effects of anal cancer treatment can linger longer than expected. Others may not appear until long after treatment is over.

Many anal cancer survivors experience problems with bowel, urinary, and sexual function.

Bowel and bladder changes

Radiation to the anus can cause tissue damage. Over time, scar tissue may form that affects how the anal muscles work.

The most commonly reported changes in bowel habits include:

- An inability to control bowel movements (fecal incontinence)
- Increase in bowel movements
- Gas (flatulence)
- Urgent need to pass stool (fecal urgency)
- Watery stool

Urinary incontinence (the inability to hold urine in the bladder) and urgency are also possible after radiation therapy for anal cancer.

There are ways to control or lessen these symptoms. Over-the-counter anti-diarrheal medicine can help with frequent and watery bowel movements, as it thickens stool.

Making changes to your diet can also help with bowel and bladder changes. Ask your care team for a list of foods that may help, as well as foods to avoid. Introducing one or more of the following may improve symptoms:

- Foods high in insoluble (not soluble) fiber
- Fiber supplements
- Psyllium-based products (like Metamucil)

There is a lot to know about oncology nutrition. Many anal cancer survivors find it helpful to talk to a dietitian who specializes in the nutritional needs of digestive system cancer survivors.

Sexual health

Treatment for anal cancer can cause changes to your sexual health and function, including:

- Difficulty getting an erection
- Reduced sex drive (libido)
- Vaginal dryness
- Pain during sex
- Narrowing and shortening of the vagina

While it may be uncomfortable to talk about sexual health, keep in mind that these side effects are common and can often be managed or lessened. Consider seeing a sexual health therapist. These health care professionals specialize in helping cancer survivors and others overcome and manage sexual side effects of cancer treatment.

Many cancer treatment centers have programs focused solely on sexual health after anal cancer treatment. Ask your provider about resources available through your cancer center that can help minimize the impact of cancer treatment on your sexual health.

Menopausal hormone therapy

The ovaries make hormones needed for menstruation and natural pregnancy. Radiation damages the ovaries, causing hormone levels to drop. This is known as premature ovarian insufficiency (POI) or radiation-induced premature menopause. It causes infertility and may also cause symptoms of menopause, including:

- Stopping of periods
- Hot flashes
- Sleeping problems
- Night sweats
- Weight gain
- Changes in mood
- Vaginal dryness

Menopausal hormone therapy may help lessen these side effects. This approach used to be called hormone replacement therapy or HRT.

Speaking with a menopause specialist or team may be helpful to determine whether menopausal hormone therapy is right for you.

Vaginal dilator therapy

Radiation therapy to the pelvic area can cause the vagina to become shorter and narrower. This is called vaginal stenosis. Vaginal stenosis can make it uncomfortable or even painful to have sex, or to have vaginal exams by a doctor.

Vaginal dilator therapy can help during and after radiation therapy. A vaginal dilator is a device used to gradually stretch or widen the vagina. Different sizes are available, as are dilator kits containing different size devices. The size of the dilator can be increased over time as the vagina lengthens and widens.

Using a dilator during radiation treatment sessions can help maintain sexual health after treatment.

Hormone changes in those assigned male at birth

Radiation damages the testicles and disrupts their ability to make hormones, such as testosterone. Symptoms of low testosterone can include:

- Reduced sex drive (libido)
- Difficulty getting an erection
- Mood changes
- Fatigue
- Increased body fat

If you are experiencing any of these symptoms, tell your care team. You may need further evaluation and management.

Pelvic floor physical therapy

The pelvic floor is a group of muscles that supports the organs of the pelvis. These muscles play a key role in bowel and bladder control and well as sexual function and arousal. There are ways to strengthen these muscles before and after treatment. This is known as pelvic floor physical therapy, and there are health care professionals who specialize in it.

Ask your care team for help finding a pelvic floor specialist in your area. Pelvic floor therapy can include at-home exercises to tighten and release the vaginal and anal muscles (Kegel exercises) as well as hands-on techniques by a physical therapist.

Ostomy care

If you have an ostomy, you may want to join an ostomy support group. Another option is to see a health care provider who specializes in ostomy care, such as an ostomy nurse.

People with ostomies can still live active lifestyles. However, it's a good idea to consult with an ostomy professional before doing any vigorous or high-intensity physical activity.

You can still lead an active lifestyle with an ostomy. However, it is a good idea to consult with an ostomy professional before doing any vigorous or high-intensity physical activity.

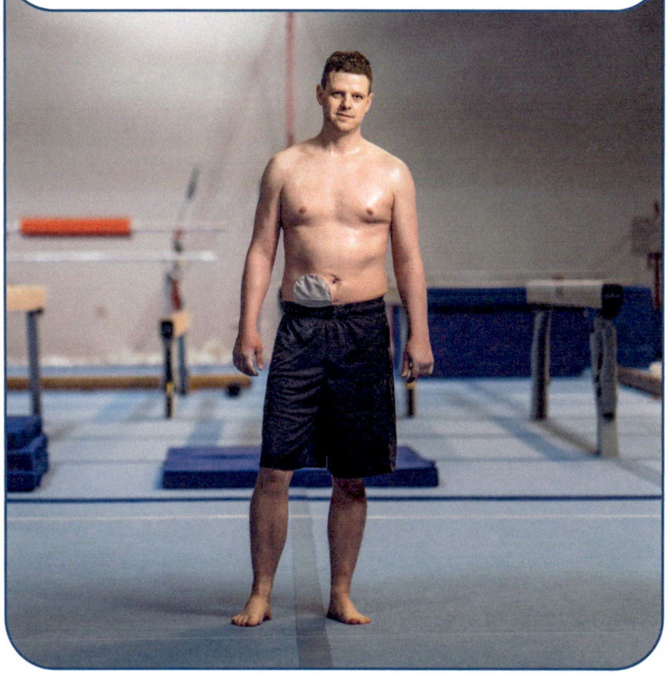

Healthy habits for cancer survivors

Follow your primary care provider's recommendations for screening for other cancers based on your age, sex, and risk level

Get other recommended health care such as blood pressure checks, hepatitis C screening, and immunizations (like the flu shot)

Eat a diet rich in plant-based foods. Limit red meat and processed foods.

Alcohol can increase the risk of some cancers. Drink little to no alcohol.

Move more, rest less. Try to exercise at a moderate intensity for at least 150 minutes per week.

Maintain a healthy weight. Tracking your weight, diet, calories, and activity levels may help you meet your goals.

Stop using tobacco. Ask your care team about options to help you quit. Counseling and medication are often options.

Radiation treatment to the pelvis increases the risk of pelvic fractures. Your provider may start checking your bone density.

Mental health and wellness

The effects of anal cancer and its treatment can be difficult to cope with. Many survivors report having an overall lower quality of life after cancer treatment.

In addition to effects on bowel, bladder, and sexual function, more general effects such as fatigue, trouble breathing, and difficulty sleeping are common. Many anal cancer survivors are also hesitant to share their diagnosis out of a fear of being judged by others. This can be isolating and distressful.

If you are anxious, distressed, depressed, or are just having trouble coping with life after cancer, you are not alone. Expect your care team to ask about your mental health. If they don't, speak up. There are resources available that can help. Social workers at your treatment site can connect you with mental health and financial resources.

For more information, see the *NCCN Guidelines for Patients: Distress During Cancer Care* at NCCN.org/patientguidelines and on the NCCN Patient Guides for Cancer app.

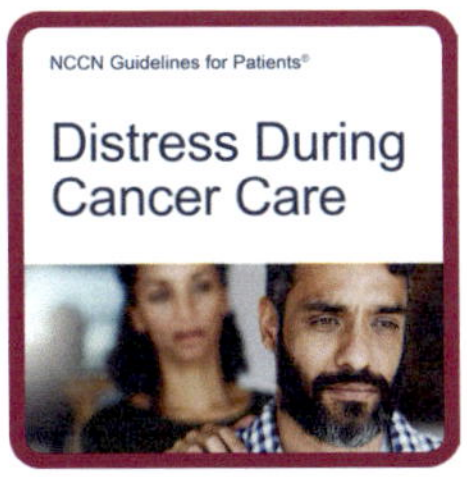

More information

For more information on cancer survivorship, the following are available at NCCN.org/patientguidelines and on the NCCN Patient Guides for Cancer app:

- *Survivorship Care for Healthy Living*
- *Survivorship Care for Cancer-Related Late and Long-Term Effects*

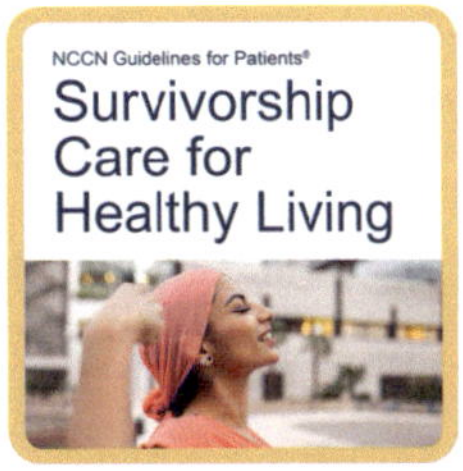

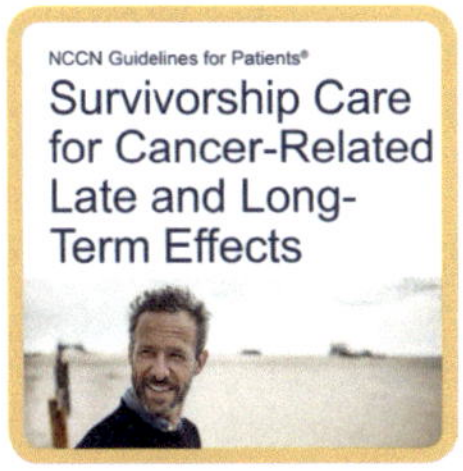

Questions to ask

- Who can I talk to about help with housing, food, and other basic needs?
- What help is available for transportation, childcare, and home care?
- Are there other services available to me and my caregivers?

5 Other resources

Want to learn more? Here's how you can get additional help.

What else to know

This book can help you improve your cancer care. It plainly explains expert recommendations and suggests questions to ask your care team. But it's not the only resource that you have.

You're welcome to receive as much information and help as you need. Many people are interested in learning more about:

- Details of their care and treatment
- Getting financial help
- Finding a care provider who is an expert in their field
- Coping with health effects

What else to do

Your health care center can help you with next steps. They often have on-site resources to help meet your needs and find answers to your questions. Health care centers can also inform you of resources in your community.

In addition to help from your providers, the resources listed in the next section provide support for many people like yourself. Look through the list and visit the provided websites to learn more about these organizations.

Where to get help

Anal Cancer Foundation
analcancerfoundation.org

CancerCare
cancercare.org

Cancer Hope Network
cancerhopenetwork.org

Cancer Survivor Care
Cancersurvivorcare.org

Colorectal Cancer Alliance
ccalliance.org

Fight Colorectal Cancer
fightcolorectalcancer.org

GRACE
Cancergrace.org

HPV Cancers Alliance
hpvalliance.org

Imerman Angels
Imermanangels.org

Love Your Buns
loveyourbuns.org

National Coalition for Cancer Survivorship
canceradvocacy.org

Triage Cancer
triagecancer.org

Words to know

abdominoperineal resection (APR)
A type of surgery that may be needed for anal cancer that doesn't respond to initial treatment or that returns after treatment. APR removes the anus, rectum, nearby cancerous lymph nodes, and other tissues. A permanent colostomy is needed.

anal canal
The small section of the large intestine that connects the rectum and the anal opening.

anal sphincter
A ring-shaped muscle around the opening of the anus that relaxes or tightens to open or close the anus.

anus
The opening at the end of the large bowel through which stool exits the body.

chemoradiation
The use of both chemotherapy and radiation therapy during the same time period (concurrently) to treat cancer. A common first treatment for anal cancer.

clinical trial
A research study using investigational treatments that may, in time, be approved by the U.S. Food and Drug Administration (FDA).

colostomy
A surgery that allows stool to leave the body after the anus is removed. The end of the bowel is attached to an opening in the surface of the abdomen. Stool is collected in a disposable bag outside of the body.

groin
The area of the body where the thigh meets the abdomen.

human papillomavirus (HPV)
A virus that affects almost everyone who has been sexually active. HPV can cause abnormal tissue growth (for example, warts) and other changes to cells. Anal cancer is almost always caused by HPV infection.

infertility
The inability to have children naturally.

inguinal lymph nodes
Lymph nodes in the groin.

intensity-modulated radiation therapy (IMRT)
A type of external radiation therapy that uses many beams of different intensities. A recommended type of radiation therapy for anal cancer.

libido
Sexual desire or the mental energy or emotion related to sex.

perianal region
The anal opening and the skin directly surrounding it. Also called the anal margin.

systemic therapy
Cancer treatment with medicines that travel through the bloodstream, reaching and affecting cells all over the body. Chemotherapy, targeted therapy, and immunotherapy are types of systemic therapy.

vaginal stenosis
A condition in which the vagina becomes narrower and shorter. The lining of the vagina may also be thinner and drier and contain scar tissue. This can cause pain during sex and pelvic exams. Vaginal stenosis is often caused by radiation therapy to the pelvis or some types of surgery.

NCCN Contributors

This patient guide is based on the NCCN Clinical Practice Guidelines in Oncology (NCCN Guidelines®) for Anal Carcinoma, Version 4.2025. It was adapted, reviewed, and published with help from the following people:

Dorothy A. Shead, MS
Senior Director
Patient Information Operations

Erin Vidic, MA
Senior Medical Writer, Patient Information

Lisa Diehl
Production Layout Artist

The NCCN Clinical Practice Guidelines in Oncology (NCCN Guidelines®) for Anal Carcinoma, Version 4.2025 were developed by the following NCCN Panel Members:

Al B. Benson, III, MD/Chair
Robert H. Lurie Comprehensive Cancer Center of Northwestern University

Alan P. Venook, MD/Vice-Chair
UCSF Helen Diller Family Comprehensive Cancer Center

Mohamed Adam, MD
UCSF Helen Diller Family Comprehensive Cancer Center

George J. Chang, MD, MS, MHCM
The University of Texas MD Anderson Cancer Center

Yi-Jen Chen, MD, PhD
City of Hope National Medical Center

Kristen K. Ciombor, MD
Vanderbilt-Ingram Cancer Center

Madison Conces, MD
Case Comprehensive Cancer Center/ University Hospitals Seidman Cancer Center and Cleveland Clinic Taussig Cancer Institute

Stacey A. Cohen, MD
Fred Hutchinson Cancer Center

Harry S. Cooper, MD
Fox Chase Cancer Center

Dustin Deming, MD
University of Wisconsin Carbone Cancer Center

Ignacio Garrido-Laguna, MD, PhD
Huntsman Cancer Institute at the University of Utah

Jean L. Grem, MD
Fred & Pamela Buffett Cancer Center

Carla Harmath, MD
The UChicago Medicine Comprehensive Cancer Center

*Paul Haste, MD
Indiana University Melvin and Bren Simon Comprehensive Cancer Center

J. Randolph Hecht, MD
UCLA Jonsson Comprehensive Cancer Center

J. Kevin Hicks, PharmD, PhD
Moffitt Cancer Center

*Sarah Hoffe, MD
Moffitt Cancer Center

Steven Hunt, MD
Siteman Cancer Center at Barnes-Jewish Hospital and Washington University School of Medicine

Hisham Hussan, MD
UC Davis Comprehensive Cancer Center

Kimberly L. Johung, MD, PhD
Yale Cancer Center/Smilow Cancer Hospital

Nora Joseph, MD
University of Michigan Rogel Cancer Center

Natalie Kirilcuk, MD
Stanford Cancer Institute

Smitha Krishnamurthi, MD
Case Comprehensive Cancer Center/ University Hospitals Seidman Cancer Center and Cleveland Clinic Taussig Cancer Institute

*Midhun Malla, MD, MS
O'Neal Comprehensive Cancer Center at UAB

Jennifer K. Maratt, MD, MS
Indiana University Melvin and Bren Simon Comprehensive Cancer Center

Wells A. Messersmith, MD
University of Colorado Cancer Center

Jeffrey Meyer, MD, MS
Johns Hopkins Kimmel Cancer Center

Jeffrey Meyerhardt, MD, MPH
Dana-Farber Brigham and Women's Cancer Center

Eric D. Miller, MD, PhD
The Ohio State University Comprehensive Cancer Center - James Cancer Hospital and Solove Research Institute

Mary F. Mulcahy, MD
Robert H. Lurie Comprehensive Cancer Center of Northwestern University

Steven Nurkin, MD, MS
Roswell Park Comprehensive Cancer Center

Hitendra Patel, MD
UC San Diego Moores Cancer Center

Katrina Pedersen, MD, MS
Mayo Clinic Comprehensive Cancer Center

Leonard Saltz, MD
Memorial Sloan Kettering Cancer Center

Charles Schneider, MD
Abramson Cancer Center at the University of Pennsylvania

David Shibata, MD
The University of Tennessee Health Science Center

* Reviewed this patient guide. For disclosures, visit NCCN.org/disclosures.

Benjamin Shogan, MD
The UChicago Medicine Comprehensive Cancer Center

Laurie Singer
DoubleLL Productions

Constantinos T. Sofocleous, MD, PhD
Memorial Sloan Kettering Cancer Center

Anna Tavakkoli, MD, MSc
UT Southwestern Simmons Comprehensive Cancer Center

Christopher G. Willett, MD
Duke Cancer Institute

Christina Wu, MD
Mayo Clinic Comprehensive Cancer Center

NCCN

Faviolla Baez-Cruz, PhD
Associate Scientist/Medical Writer

Lisa Gurski, PhD
Senior Manager, Licensed Clinical Content

Frankie Jones
Guidelines Coordinator

We want your feedback!

Our goal is to provide helpful and easy-to-understand information on cancer. Take our survey to let us know what we got right and what we could do better. NCCN.org/patients/feedback

NCCN Cancer Centers

Abramson Cancer Center
at the University of Pennsylvania
Philadelphia, Pennsylvania
800.789.7366 • pennmedicine.org/cancer

Case Comprehensive Cancer Center/
University Hospitals Seidman Cancer Center and
Cleveland Clinic Taussig Cancer Institute
Cleveland, Ohio
UH Seidman Cancer Center
800.641.2422 • uhhospitals.org/services/cancer-services
CC Taussig Cancer Institute
866.223.8100 • my.clevelandclinic.org/departments/cancer
Case CCC
216.844.8797 • case.edu/cancer

City of Hope National Medical Center
Duarte, California
800.826.4673 • cityofhope.org

Dana-Farber/Brigham and Women's Cancer Center |
Mass General Cancer Center
Boston, Massachusetts
877.442.3324 • youhaveus.org
617.726.5130 • massgeneral.org/cancer-center

Duke Cancer Institute
Durham, North Carolina
888.275.3853 • dukecancerinstitute.org

Fox Chase Cancer Center
Philadelphia, Pennsylvania
888.369.2427 • foxchase.org

Fred & Pamela Buffett Cancer Center
Omaha, Nebraska
402.559.5600 • unmc.edu/cancercenter

Fred Hutchinson Cancer Center
Seattle, Washington
206.667.5000 • fredhutch.org

Huntsman Cancer Institute at the University of Utah
Salt Lake City, Utah
800.824.2073 • healthcare.utah.edu/huntsmancancerinstitute

Indiana University Melvin and Bren Simon
Comprehensive Cancer Center
Indianapolis, Indiana
888.600.4822 • www.cancer.iu.edu

Johns Hopkins Kimmel Cancer Center
Baltimore, Maryland
410.955.8964
www.hopkinskimmelcancercenter.org

Mayo Clinic Comprehensive Cancer Center
Phoenix/Scottsdale, Arizona
Jacksonville, Florida
Rochester, Minnesota
480.301.8000 • Arizona
904.953.0853 • Florida
507.538.3270 • Minnesota
mayoclinic.org/cancercenter

Memorial Sloan Kettering Cancer Center
New York, New York
800.525.2225 • mskcc.org

Moffitt Cancer Center
Tampa, Florida
888.663.3488 • moffitt.org

O'Neal Comprehensive Cancer Center at UAB
Birmingham, Alabama
800.822.0933 • uab.edu/onealcancercenter

Robert H. Lurie Comprehensive Cancer Center
of Northwestern University
Chicago, Illinois
866.587.4322 • cancer.northwestern.edu

Roswell Park Comprehensive Cancer Center
Buffalo, New York
877.275.7724 • roswellpark.org

Siteman Cancer Center at Barnes-Jewish Hospital
and Washington University School of Medicine
St. Louis, Missouri
800.600.3606 • siteman.wustl.edu

St. Jude Children's Research Hospital/
The University of Tennessee Health Science Center
Memphis, Tennessee
866.278.5833 • stjude.org
901.448.5500 • uthsc.edu

Stanford Cancer Institute
Stanford, California
877.668.7535 • cancer.stanford.edu

The Ohio State University Comprehensive Cancer Center -
James Cancer Hospital and Solove Research Institute
Columbus, Ohio
800.293.5066 • cancer.osu.edu

The UChicago Medicine Comprehensive Cancer Center
Chicago, Illinois
773.702.1000 • uchicagomedicine.org/cancer

The University of Texas MD Anderson Cancer Center
Houston, Texas
844.269.5922 • mdanderson.org

UC Davis Comprehensive Cancer Center
Sacramento, California
916.734.5959 • 800.770.9261
health.ucdavis.edu/cancer

UC San Diego Moores Cancer Center
La Jolla, California
858.822.6100 • cancer.ucsd.edu

UCLA Jonsson Comprehensive Cancer Center
Los Angeles, California
310.825.5268 • uclahealth.org/cancer

UCSF Helen Diller Family
Comprehensive Cancer Center
San Francisco, California
800.689.8273 • cancer.ucsf.edu

University of Colorado Cancer Center
Aurora, Colorado
720.848.0300 • coloradocancercenter.org

University of Michigan Rogel Cancer Center
Ann Arbor, Michigan
800.865.1125 • rogelcancercenter.org

University of Wisconsin Carbone Cancer Center
Madison, Wisconsin
608.265.1700 • uwhealth.org/cancer

UT Southwestern Simmons
Comprehensive Cancer Center
Dallas, Texas
214.648.3111 • utsouthwestern.edu/simmons

Vanderbilt-Ingram Cancer Center
Nashville, Tennessee
877.936.8422 • vicc.org

Yale Cancer Center/Smilow Cancer Hospital
New Haven, Connecticut
855.4.SMILOW • yalecancercenter.org

share with us.

Take our survey and help make the NCCN Guidelines for Patients better for everyone!

NCCN.org/patients/comments

Index

Made in United States
Cleveland, OH
31 March 2026

35186511R10029